THOUSANDS OF YEARS AGO . . .

. . . a form of molasses was used in India as both food and medicine. It was used to purify the blood, prevent rheumatic and bile disorders, as well as to nourish the body.

Today's molasses has all the same health-giving properties as its ancient Eastern ancestor.

This highly informative book exposes the harmful effects of eating refined sugar. It reveals exactly why molasses is better for the entire system, tastes better—and show exactly how to use it *deliciously* in your diet!

Here is a guide to help yourself by working *with* Nature, not against her!

Everything You Want to Know About

MOLASSES

Natural Food—
Natural Remedy

P. E. NORRIS

Preface by CARLSON WADE

THE PYRAMID HEALTHFUL LIVING SERIES

Pyramid Books • New York

NOTE TO READERS: This special American edition has been carefully edited to make it easily understood by our readers. British spellings, sources, language differentials have been Americanized. There are some idiomatic phrases and specifics that are so traditionally British they had to remain, so that the meanings would be kept as the author intended them to be. The text of the book is now carefully Americanized to offer you healthful knowledge that bridges the language gap.

EVERYTHING YOU WANT TO KNOW ABOUT MOLASSES

A PYRAMID BOOK
Published by arrangement with Thorsons Publishers Limited

© P. E. Norris, 1960
Preface Copyright © 1972 by Carlson Wade

All Rights Reserved

Pyramid Healthful Living Edition published March, 1972

Printed in the United States of America

ISBN 0-7225-0005x

Pyramid Books are published by Pyramid Communications, Inc. Its trademarks, consisting of the word "Pyramid" and the portrayal of a pyramid, are registered in the United States Patent Office.

PYRAMID COMMUNICATIONS, INC.
919 Third Avenue
New York, New York 10022, U.S.A.

CONTENTS

PREFACE
by
CARLSON WADE

For those who want to satisfy a sweet tooth, yet want to keep away from sugar, this book is an excursion into the world of healthfully delicious sweeteners. In particular, the book tells of molasses—the sugar that nourishes. It tells just how molasses is made, why it is superior to other sweeteners, why it is able to build health while catering to the urge to have something sweet.

The author has done a marvelous research job into the actual making of molasses and the reasons why it can be used with comparative safety and health. He makes no pretenses about sugar. He says that it does give energy—but "no more energy than we should get from foods that contain the bonus of vitamins, minerals and protein." He offers molasses as such a food!

P. E. Norris tells why white sugar is harmful, how it can lead to overweight, impair the teeth, create glandular disturbances, contribute to diabetes, and upset the delicate mechanism of the hormonal system.

Then he offers the molasses side of the sweet story. He provides a special set of charts to back up his discovery that molasses is a treasure of minerals, vitamins and other substances that work to build health—while you enjoy the sweet taste.

He is honest when he says that to eat molasses at every meal is NOT a good idea. "Nor is it a good idea to eat any one food at every meal." Instead, he suggests that you eat just about a full teaspoon of molasses at one meal a day. He then gives you a delicious breakfast that includes molasses. He says that this will "make an excellent breakfast to start the day." I took his word for it, prepared such a breakfast and found myself facing the day with energy and mental alertness that made me feel wonderfully "young" until nightfall. Molasses is certainly a "morning energizer," and P. E. Norris is to be commended for having written this helpful book.

He asserts, "You must work *with* Nature and not *against* it." Showing how molasses can be one part of health boosting, he offers programs for improving health with molasses as a starter. The special recipe section is a classic treasure in itself, especially the various milk shakes and beverages using molasses. Just one sip and you'll become a molasses lover and feel healthier for it, too. Thank you, Mr. Norris, for this book!

Everything You Want to Know About Molasses by P. E. Norris is a sweet treasure of natural health tips.

MOLASSES

AS MOLASSES is a product of the sugar cane, it would be as well to say something about the cane, the parent from which both molasses and sugar come.

The word "sugar" comes from the Sanskrit "sakara," which is also the root from which many other words meaning "sugar" are derived, such as: sukkar (Arabic), azucar (Spanish), acucar (Portuguese), zucchero (Italian), sucre (French), zucker (German), zocker (Flemish), suiker (Dutch), socker (Swedish), sachar (Russian), szukor (Hungarian), and shakar or sheker (Persian).

The word "candy" is derived from the Sanskrit "khanda."

Sugar cane thrives only in the tropics, for the plant needs hot sun, but the sugar beet, from which beet-sugar and beet-molasses is extracted, thrives in temperate climates.

History of Sugar Cane

The cane was grown and sweet products made from its sap in ancient times in India, China, Malaya and some of the islands in the Pacific. For centuries India produced and ate a dark brown sugar, but white sugar came in all probability from China, which was the first country to produce a paler product. This was known in India as "cheenee," or "a product of China."

Unless proof, documentary or archeological, is unearthed, we will never know for certain who first manufactured sugar.

The first known reference to sugar occurs in the *Atharva Veda* of the Hindus, *circa* 500 B.C. Two hundred years later when Nearchos and Onesicritos, two of Alexander the Great's officers, visited the

Indus Valley, they wrote (according to Von Lippman's translation): "In India there is said to be a reed which yields honey without the help of bees; also that it yields an intoxicating drink even though the plant does not bear fruit."

Those at home were skeptical for it sounded like a tall traveler's tale. But eventually, about eight centuries later, sugar reached the Mediterranean countries where, owing to its excessive cost, it was eaten by only the wealthy. Ultimately it came to England where, we are told, in 1262 Edward I ordered sugar for the royal household; and about fifty years later a considerable quantity of sugar was imported by nobles and other rich men at a cost of 1 shilling 9½ pence a pound, the equivalent of which today would be about £10.

By another 300 years the Spanish and Portuguese had planted the cane in Madeira, the Canaries, Cape Verde Islands, and West Africa, and on his second voyage in 1493 Columbus carried cane roots to the West Indies, where a vast new industry sprang into being. But it wasn't until 1788 that the sugar cane was first grown in Queensland, Australia, now a flourishing center of the industry.

The growth of the sugar industry in the United Kingdom has been remarkable. In 1750 some fifty refineries produced 30,000 tons a year; today 2,500,000 tons are refined annually.

Why S-U-G-A-R is pronounced as it is no one knows, but it is this that impelled an American expert on semantics to turn to Bernard Shaw and remark, "Do you realize, Mr. Shaw, that 'sugar' is the only word in the English language where 's' is pronounced as 'sh'?"

"Sure," agreed G.B.S.

Sugar cane is technically a grass—one of about 300 kinds. Bamboo is another.

Sugar cane grows to a height of 12–15 feet. The stalk is from one to two inches in diameter and consists mainly of soft fiber which when ripe is filled with rich, sweet juice.

Manufacturing Processes

To manufacture sugar the cane is crushed between steel rollers which have been sprinkled with water to help free the juice. At this stage (varying with the quality of the cane) the juice contains 8–21 per cent sugar, 2½ per cent impurities, and the remainder water.

In a modern factory the cane goes through as many as five sets of rollers, until no more juice can be extracted. The pulp, known as bagasse, is used to feed furnaces for boiling the juice, and the surplus is returned to the fields as humus.

In order to get rid of the impurities a little lime is added to the juice and it is heated again; the impurities then coagulate and settle as "mud." This "mud" is filtered off and used as fertilizer on the fields.

In the past it was merely dumped in some out-of-the-way spot and stank; or a river flowed by and the "mud" was drained into it. Many years ago, however, a local health officer said that the water in a river where "mud" was dumped was being polluted, so the owner of the sugar factory dumped it in an unused field where it grew and grew, decomposed and attracted hordes of flies. This annoyed the manager's wife who remembered that one of the assistants had expressed the opinion that "mud" could be used. "Get rid of the stuff," she told him; "we don't mind what you do with it."

He commandeered half a dozen trucks, loaded them with "mud," trundled it to the poorest farm in the district and sprayed it on the land. As a result the farm, which was yielding a mere 4,000 tons of sugar a year, increased its output to 24,000! This made everyone sit up, and ever since "mud" has been regarded as a valuable by-product.

After the "mud" has been filtered off the juice is again boiled in steam-heated vacuum pans until a "massecuite" or mixture of sugar crystals and syrup is formed. The massecuite is spun in centrifugal machines to separate the crystals (cane sugar) from the residual syrup (molasses).

The raw sugar is then sent to the refineries. Water is added to the molasses and it is boiled again. This time crystals lighter in color are formed and there is still some syrup left over. Each time the process takes place the crystals take on a lighter hue.

The process is the same whether the juice comes from the cane or the beet, for chemically there is no difference between them; but as far as smell is concerned there is no comparison. Cane sugar has a rich appetizing aroma like old-fashioned toffee, whereas a good sniff of beet sugar makes one reel back. No one in his senses would eat beet sugar if he could buy the product of the cane for the same price, but so emasculated are people's tastes today that many don't realize there is any difference!

Sugar cane juice varies in color from gray to dark green, depending on the quality of the cane from which it is expressed and the soil in which it is grown. In solution it contains about 70–72 per cent water, 1–2.8 per cent protein, 8–21 per cent sugar consisting of sucrose, dextrose and levulose; 5 per cent ash made up of silica, potash, soda, lime, magnesia, iron, phosphoric and sulfuric acids, and chlorine; and nitrogenous substances, such as albuminoids, amides, amino acids, nitric acid, ammonia and xanthin bodies. In cane juice there is also 0.6 per cent fat and wax, pectin (gums) and organic acids.

In India one doubts whether the juice of the cane was ever manufactured into the paler crystals which appear on our tables until after British rule. But Indians have always manufactured "gur" or jaggery, a substance made from the juice of either the cane or the palm, and varying in hue from dark brown to cream. Jaggery is still widely used in Indian cookery and many delicious and nutritious sweets are made with it, and all over India it is sold in plates the shape of a discus.

Sugar, molasses, jaggery, sugar candy and toddy (an alcoholic beverage) are also manufactured from the sap of palm trees—palmyra palm, date palm, coconut palm and sago palm, and in India palmyra and date account for 97 per cent of the jaggery made.

The trees are tapped and the juice collected in large earthenware vessels. It is then treated in exactly the same way as sugar cane juice or the juice of the beet; and the jaggery and molasses from these sources is very similar in composition to that made from cane or beet.

Palm Sap Products

In India the industry producing jaggery is a cottage industry, and though only a very small percentage of palms are tapped for juice to be made into jaggery (about 10,000,000), more than 170,000 tons of jaggery and cane products are made from their juices.

Jaggery is a health food, rich in mineral salts and infinitely more palatable than the nicest-tasting molasses. The government intends to control the industry, and when this is done the product will doubtless be exported to Europe and America.

According to Dr. S. C. Roy of the Indian Central Sugarcane Committee, jaggery is both a food and a medicine. It acts as a mild laxative, has a greater warming effect than sugar, and is sweeter. Throughout India it is fed to both mothers and cows during lactation and is prescribed for many ailments in the indigenous system of medicine (kaviraj).

The *Sasrutha Sanhita* (chapter 45, sloka 146),

compiled 2,500 years ago, states that slightly old jaggery purifies the blood, prevents rheumatic and bile disorders, and is a nourishing food of high order.

The difference between white sugar on one hand, and either cane molasses and jaggery on the other, is that white sugar is manufactured by clarifying cane juice under chemical treatment and concentrating it so that the crystals may be separated from the mother sap by mechanical means.

White sugar contains 99 per cent sucrose and a negligible amount of moisture and so-called "impurities."

"Gur (jaggery)," according to Dr. Roy, "is the whole cane juice or the sap of palm trees in its natural state in a concentrated form. Except for a small change during the boiling process it contains all the constituents of the mother juice, and its composition is essentially the same as the pure juice, though the proportion of the constituents varies according to the variety of the cane and the method of manufacture.

"Generally speaking it consists of: sucrose 65–85 per cent, invert sugar 10–15 per cent, ash 2–5 per cent, moisture 3–6 per cent."

All this can be very confusing to the layman. He picks up, for instance, an excellent little book like *The Story of Sugar* by L. A. G. Strong, who says that when he asked a Harley Street physician what sugar was, the medical man replied, "Vital energy. A primal source of life."

Strong put the same question to a Hindu philosopher who gave this answer: "The life-giving energy of the sun."

Then he heard the General Manager of a West Indian sugar company lecture to boys at a public school, and this is what that authority told them: "The energy derived from the sun for the formation of sugar in the cane is preserved and released when the sugar crystals are eaten; it is therefore, in effect, crystallized sunlight."

And then the layman might pick up Brigadier Bernard Fergusson's book, *Beyond the Chindwin*, and read that the men under Fergusson's command were on one occasion so exhausted that they could not speak; but when given a kind of sugar-fudge to eat they "spoke with tongues."

All of which gives him the impression that sugar —any sugar; ordinary white sugar—is a kind of manna from heaven; that it contains all sorts of rejuvenating and strengthening properties, whereas in actual fact nothing could be farther from the truth.

As a medium that imparts no other flavor to food than sweetness, WHITE, REFINED sugar is without a rival, for Demerara, "pieces," Barbados and Muscavados each has a distinctive flavor, and "foot sugar" very much so. It is like black treacle.

Constituents other than sucrose, which were present in the original juice, are thrown out in molasses (or jaggery). White sugar is therefore a PURE (*i.e.*, unmixed with any other substance), simple carbohydrate of the disaccharide class, so that before it can be assimilated it must be broken down into a monosaccharide.

John Yudkin, Professor of Nutrition, London University, wrote recently, "Much of our present dietary arises from the fact that 200 years ago Man learned how to isolate sugar.

"When your great-great-great-grandfather wanted something sweet, he ate fruits or berries.

"Today if we want something sweet, nine times out of ten we take chocolate, sweets, ice cream, cakes or a sweetened drink which may taste just like fruit juice, but isn't.

"As these manufactured foods and drinks contain little or nothing in the way of nutrients except sugar, we are fooling Nature.

"True, sugar gives us energy; but no more energy than we should get from foods that contain the bonus of vitamins, minerals and protein. My view is that Man becomes addicted to sugar as easily as he does to tobacco or cocaine. Today we eat as much sugar in two weeks as our great-great-great-grandfathers ate in a year."

Now all this may seem very confusing and complicated.

You wanted to learn about molasses and I seem to have side-tracked you onto the subject of sugar.

But unless you know what molasses is and why it differs from sugar you'll never be satisfied in your own mind that molasses is good for you, whereas white sugar is not.

The fact that you've persisted so far is a tribute to your desire to learn, and your tenacity. In an age when nearly everyone wishes to be spoon-fed, you are willing to use your intelligence and reasoning power.

So let's go on to the next chapter.

WHY WHITE SUGAR IS HARMFUL AND MOLASSES NOURISHES

ADVERTISEMENTS in newspapers, magazines and on TV tell us every day that SUGAR IS GOOD FOR YOU; that sugar gives you energy; that sugar is essential for growing children.

All this is strictly true. But what the advertisements fail to tell you is that white, refined sugar, from which almost all sugar-laden commodities are made, is *NOT* good for you. Taken in all but the smallest amounts, it is harmful.

You don't have to take my word for it. On November 17, 1955, *The British Medical Journal* stated: "The purpose of food is to nourish, and substances intended for Man's consumption— proteins, carbohydrates, fats, vitamins, salts and catalysts are in Nature associated with each other and other substances in such a way as to render them acceptable to the human economy. If in his presumptuous ignorance Man tampers with these substances by cooking them, concentrating them, and refining them he may retain the main proximate principle, but he deprives it of the associates which render it tolerable to the human digestive organs. If, for example, he concentrates a bison into a beaker he may get the major portion of the protein, but he will get very little else save, perchance, a stomach ache. That is an extreme case.

"That of sugar is almost as extreme, though not quite. Pure sugar ($C_{12}H_{22}O_{11}$) is a very irritating substance, as may be seen from the eczema which is so apt to trouble the hands and arms of grocers who handle it.

"In its natural state as in the cane or in fruit, sugar is associated with various substances which dilute and mitigate the irritant properties of the pure chemical. The reason why soft *brown sugar is more digestible than white* is that the brown is less refined than the white; *the browner it is, the cruder and more digestible.*"

In cases of illness refined sugar may cause irritation to the stomach if taken undiluted and in substantial quantities. That is why sick people are told to take glucose, though it is not meant for those who are healthy and whose digestive organs function perfectly. You will see why later in this chapter.

No one who knows anything about food and its relation to health will recommend white sugar. In *You're The Doctor*, Victor Heiser, M.D., says: "No sweet course would be included in my ideal diet. If I wish to be on top form I take no refined sugar.

"Too much sugar and too much fat, the other great energy food, usually produce overweight, which predisposes to diabetes. Although it may have no connection, it is worthy of note that the great increase of this disease has occurred among the wrong eaters and has also been coincidental with the great increase in sugar and fat consumption. . . ."

Heiser is only one of scores of medical men and dental surgeons who condemn the use of refined sugar. Professor R. H. A. Plimmer of London University writes: "Barker and Hoffman's statistics show that cancer and diabetes are increasing all over the world, and at the same time there is a corresponding increase in the consumption of white cereals and refined sugar. Such a diet, *with its shortage of vitamin B*, is known to be responsible for the preliminary troubles which may culminate in cancer and diabetes.

"We ought to eat the *whole cane sugar* or the whole beet, or sweet fruit, but not the extracted sugar. We need the residues which are discarded [from refined sugar]. . . . Sugar forms no part of the diet of the Indian hill tribe of the state of Hunza whom Dr. McCarrison describes as living on natural foods and having perfect health and physique."

We also know that Stefansson, the famous explorer, said that primitive Eskimos had no knowledge of purgatives, nor need of them. But as soon as the white trader came along with refined sugar and white flour, with no bulky acid fruits to balance their diet, they became the most constipated people on earth.

The British used to consume 17 pounds of sugar per head in 1840; in 1953 the consumption had gone up to 100 pounds a head. In America even more refined sugar is eaten, but according to *Family Doctor* (May 1953) American medical men claim that merely by cutting down the amount of white flour and refined sugar eaten they can also reduce considerably the susceptibility to colds.

Sugar is condemned by the heads of the dental profession. Dr. J. Sim Wallace says in his book *Oral Hygiene*, "Sugar is so highly refined that we may almost say that it is not a food but a pure chemical product produced in quantity for the destruction of the teeth."

At the end of the eighteenth century sugar refining processes were not as efficient as today and the sugar eaten in Britain was soft and dark; puddings were made with black treacle or molasses, between which there is very little difference.

In his very interesting book, *A West-India Fortune*, Richard Pares tells us that the brewers and distillers in the eighteenth century demanded sugar, and ultimately Parliament forbade its use in West Indian distilleries. "This brought the distillers into the market for molasses and forced the consumers to buy brown sugar instead, incidentally encouraging the sugar refiners, who turned out molasses as a by-product."

White Sugar Cannot Nourish

There are many kinds of sugar: glucose, fructose, sucrose, lactose, maltose, levulose, mannose, xylose, and galactose, all of which are sweet and soluble in water. All come from different sources—but you don't have to worry your head about them.

What you must bear in mind is that sweetness alone, though pleasant to the palate, has no nutritive effect whatever, unless some article of food value has been added to the sweet matter—such as cocoa in chocolate; the fat and milk in toffee; or the vitamins and minerals found in their natural state in molasses, dark sugars, and fruits. Saccharin, though infinitely sweeter than refined sugar, is no relation of sugar and has not one iota of food value.

White sugar, with which most people lace their coffee and tea, has only calorific value and imparts heat and temporary energy to the body. It does not nourish unless combined with some other food.

Fruit sugar, however, such as is found in raisins, sultanas, currants, dates, figs, and in fresh fruits, is rich in minerals; and in the case of fresh fruits, of vitamins as well. Into this category may be placed honey, molasses, black treacle and jaggery.

Indian scientists have done a great deal of research with sugar, molasses and jaggery, and Dr. H. G. Biswas wrote in *Science and Industry* (1938) that both cane molasses and date palm jaggery contain appreciable quantities of vitamins B_1 and B_2 and are superior in every way to white sugar. "Factory" white sugar, which is much darker than that sold for table use, contains no calcium or phosphates; but molasses and jaggery do. In every 100 milligrams of white sugar there were 0.97 grams of iron and 0.086 of copper, whereas the figures for jaggery and molasses were 11.36 and 0.51 and 15.66 and 0.57 respectively.

Experiments were carried out with young rats each weighing approximately 38 grams. They were divided into three groups and each group was fed on milk. One group, however, was given an addition of open pan (not refined) white sugar, the second jaggery and the third molasses. At the end of seven months the average weight of the first group was 125, the second 144 and the third 150 grams. Had refined sugar, such as is found on our tables, been used, the difference would have been even more marked.

Now a word about glucose. Advertisements everywhere inform us that this or that product contains glucose—as if it were a virtue! The makers usually add that not only does glucose provide energy, but it provides "instant energy," because it needs no digesting and goes straight into the bloodstream.

All this is perfectly true; but the implication that a food that needs no digesting is superior to one that does is quite wrong.

Why should Nature provide digestive organs if there were no need for them? Arguing on the same lines, why not extract the nation's teeth and feed everyone on pap. That would certainly simplify life.

In his book, *Sports Injuries*, Dr. Christopher Woodward, Honorary Consultant to the British Olympic teams in 1948 and 1952, writes: "The best forms of sugar in order of digestibility are brown sugar, honey, treacle and white sugar. *I do not recommend glucose because it usually gives fit men and women indigestion.* It is, so to speak, a predigested form of sugar, and whereas it is all right for old ladies who cannot digest sugar for themselves, it is not the sort of thing that a normally fit person should need to take."

Glucose is also condemned in an article by Margaret Lamb, L.D.S., in *The British Dental Journal*, October 21, 1958, who says: "For the body to use carbohydrate successfully *vitamin B must be present* and, if it is not supplied with the food as it is in natural sugar, *then the vitamin is absorbed from the body's storage depots.*

"Quite often on the labels of sweet jars, certain

jams and jellies and invalid drinks, you read that the product is made from glucose—as though that were a virtue. Glucose is a synthetic product made by treating corn starch with hydrochloric acid or sulphuric acid, neutralizing the resultant syrup with calcium carbonate and decolorizing with carbon or bone black. According to Leo, the American nutritionist, *glucose is the only known sugar to cause diabetes in test animals.*"

So much for the advertisements.

The idea that glucose in a drink will provide any appreciable amount of energy is utter nonsense. According to a report of the Food Standards Committee submitted to the Minister of Health (*Manchester Guardian*, Feb. 25, 1959): "Whatever form of carbohydrate sweetening is used in soft drinks, it will not contribute more than a fraction of a normal person's energy requirement."

The report discusses the merits of sucrose, glucose and "liquid glucose" as sources of energy and states that whereas glucose, but not sucrose, administered intravenously (in a vein) can be of immense benefit to *patients suffering from a variety of conditions*, it is a fallacy to infer that glucose is a more desirable form of energy than when taken through the mouth. The Report continues:

"It is to be doubted whether there is any advantage in presenting to the human being a drink which contains a sugar which is a little more rapidly metabolized than others, but if such a sugar be deemed to be of value the balance of evidence suggests that sucrose might be chosen rather than glucose or the products of the partial hydrolysis of starch which is found in commercial 'liquid glucose.' "

I have dilated on this theme in order to dispel once and for all the notion that so-called commercial "fruit drinks" are of any appreciable value. At most they contain 25 per cent fruit juice; often none at all—merely water, glucose and chemicals!

During the past thirty years I have studied dozens of books on food and dietetics but in only three (except those written in India) can I find anything but the barest reference to either black treacle or molasses. And where we are told that molasses is good for you, or that it either cures or alleviates this condition or that, no reasons are advanced.

I happen to be one of those unpleasant, skeptical persons who likes to know why, and few books on the subject set out to satisfy this urge for knowledge as far as molasses is concerned. So I have been compelled to ferret and dig out the information I am giving you.

There is, of course, a fair amount of literature to explain why molasses is good for animals and the United Molasses Company, which sells crude molasses for cattle, sheep, pigs and chickens, has had its product analyzed and can tell you just what it contains and why it is good for farmyard stock.

And if for animals, why not humans?

Those who in childhood lived on farms thirty years ago sometimes sneaked round to the barn where the molasses was stored in a barrel, pulled out the bung, allowed a thick, green-black dollop to flow sluggishly onto one finger and then shut off the supply. Into the mouth this bitter-sweet morsel was popped and off the child would run.

Dirty this treacle or molasses might have been but it did no one a bit of harm and when one's pocket-money was exhausted, was a fine standby. It fattened pigs and it put pounds on children, too, but as long as they didn't sit around getting fat, it was good for them.

It always seems odd to me that prize farm animals and racehorses are fed more scientifically and with greater care than humans; they are given only such food as will make them stronger, tougher and more resistant to disease. Or perhaps it's not so odd, because such animals, either dead or alive, if in prime condition, represent money to their owners.

Humans can maltreat themselves and no one is a penny the worse off, and as the most important commodity in the world today appears to be money and not human welfare, no government will go out of its way to tell people how to look after themselves, unless it is in the government interest.

One is cynical about government propaganda. Only recently, because of the enormous capital sunk in chicken farming, the government put up an "expert" to assure the people that small eggs had every bit as much nutriment as big eggs; and that eggs and chickens reared in batteries were the equal, nutritionally, of free-ranging chickens and the eggs they laid.

What you want to do is to think, ask questions, read. Don't be content to sit in front of the TV set and swallow all the garbage that is poured out. Sift and find out the truth for yourself.

No government body will advise you to discard refined sugar and make puddings and cakes with brown sugar, treacle or molasses.

The Saccharide Family

The simplest sugars are monosaccharides—from "mono," meaning "one." They consist of six atoms of carbon combined with six molecules of water; for those with a smattering of chemistry, one molecule of monosaccharide is written thus: $C_6(H_2O_6)$ or $C_6H_{12}O_6$.

If two molecules of a monosaccharide, or two molecules of two different saccharides combine, they form a disaccharide, from "di," meaning "two."

If a number of monosaccharides combine they form a polysaccharide, from "poly," meaning "many."

Monosaccharides occur in fruits, some vegetables, honey, golden syrup, and of course, glucose.

Disaccharides are cane sugar, beet sugar, palm or date sugar (jaggery) and lactose and milk sugar. Molasses, of course, comes into this category.

In the polysaccharide class we have flour, macaroni, biscuits, breakfast cereals, potatoes, pulses, cakes, bread, some nuts, etc.

Monosaccharides need no digestion and pass straight into the bloodstream, but as already explained, there is no advantage in this except in the cases of invalids.

Nature has provided your body with enzymes or ferments which act upon di- and polysaccharides and break them down into monosaccharides, so that they can be digested. If you don't use your digestive organs they become flabby and sluggish like unused muscles.

Moreover, Nature provided you with a set of teeth and—one hopes—the desire to use them. The first process in the digestion of all carbohydrate takes place in the mouth. As the teeth chew and crush carbohydrate the tongue helps it to mix with an enzyme called ptyalin, which is released and helps digestion. If food is not properly chewed, complete digestion does not take place, and if chewing is neglected over a fair period digestive troubles set in.

Composition of Molasses

Having explained why refined sugar is harmful I hope now to show why molasses and black treacle, which is an allied product, are beneficial.

Crude molasses, *as supplied for animals*, consists of 48 per cent total sugars (expressed as invert); 12.19 per cent sugar other than carbohydrate; 4.81 per cent crude protein; 12.44 per cent mineral matter; and 22.56 per cent water.

Its value lies chiefly in the mineral matter and vitamins, and the mineral matter consists of:

Silica (SiO_2)	3.700
Iron oxide (Fe_2O_3)	0.500
Lime (CaO)	13.550
Magnesium Oxide (MgO)	9.400
Potassium Oxide (K_2O)	38.650
Sodium Oxide (Na_2O)	1.085
Sulphur Trioxide (SO_3)	12.550
Phosphorus Pentoxide (P_2O_5)	1.830
Chlorine (Cl)	20.370
Carbon Dioxide (CO_2) by difference	3.285
	104.595
Less Oxygen equivalent of chlorine	4.595
	100.000

The vitamin content of crude molasses in milligrams per pound is:

Aneurin (called thiamine in U.S.A.)	0.4
Riboflavin (also called vitamin G or B_2)	1.0
Nicotinic acid (called niacin in U.S.A.)	21.3
Pantothenic acid	19.5
Choline	290.0

All these belong to the vitamin B group, or the B complex.

Below are figures for the composition of blackstrap molasses.

Moisture	24.58
Mineral matter	8.32
Levulose	8.76
Cane sugar	30.08
Dextrose	13.06
Other carbohydrates and organic matter	13.20
	100.00

The mineral matter consists of:

Magnesia	0.3600
Calcium phosphate, etc.	5.3354
Sodium salts	0.3600
Potassium salts	2.2400
Iron	0.0200
Copper	0.0040
Lead	0.0005
Arsenic	0.0001
	8.3200

The organic matter consists of:

Gummy matter	2.70
Nitrogenous bodies	1.06
Organic acids	3.20
Caramel and other products of decomposition made during manufacture of raw sugar crystals	6.24
	13.20

Beware of any crude or other molasses to which the sulfur dioxide is added as a preservative. In the U.S.A. this is banned by law.

Molasses is a good laxative food, but one doubts whether it is a better natural laxative than bran, and certainly not as effective as beetroot. A whole beet eaten with salad is the most effective of natural laxatives and will cure all but the most stubborn types of constipation.

To eat molasses at every meal is NOT a good idea. Nor is it a good idea to eat any one food at every meal; even bread, though some feel lost without bread. Though easily digested, there are some digestions that may not be able to tolerate a continuous intake of molasses or treacle.

If you are going to eat molasses regularly, do not eat more than a full teaspoon at any one meal. Two dessertspoons of wheat germ, one of bran, a teaspoon of molasses or black treacle and either warm or cold milk make an excellent breakfast to start the day.

At night take a teaspoon of molasses or treacle in warm water or milk.

More may nauseate one. If you doubt this, try it and find out for yourself. You may be able to tolerate a great deal more molasses or treacle than I can.

There are innumerable ways in which both can be used and recipes are given at the end of this volume.

WHY YOUR BODY NEEDS MINERALS

THE chief value of molasses lies in the fact that it is rich in minerals, vitamins of the B family and perhaps some principle as yet not discovered by Man. There are foods which, one is sure, contain nutriment in some form which we as yet know nothing about. The date must be one.

Books on food and dietetics often unwittingly give erroneous impressions. They speak about vitamins and minerals being "protective" foods; they describe proteins as body builders and carbohydrates as producers of energy. Yet, fat is as great an energy producer as carbohydrate, and without vitamin C, for instance, the body would deteriorate rapidly.

Because of this misleading information those who think they are weak are apt to stuff with proteins and as a result contract digestive troubles and suffer from acidity. If they feel they lack energy they devour carbohydrates and put on excessive weight.

The various classes of food are complementary. The person who studies diet (not mere book learning) and experiments with his own body soon learns how to balance his diet and eat what suits him, and how much.

One cannot ignore food in any of these groups and continue in perfect health; a proportion of each group is needed.

The body contains many mineral elements, all to be found in their natural state in fruits, vegetables, nuts, legumes, milk and meat—also in water. They are loosely referred to as "mineral salts" because some of them are not present in food in the shape of inorganic salts. As those with even a smattering of chemistry know, a chemical salt is a compound produced by the reaction between an acid and a base (alkali).

We don't as yet know the purpose or function of all the minerals in the body—there are nearly forty!—some in comparatively large quantities; some in mere traces. We know a good deal, however, about the major minerals like iron, calcium, phosphorus, etc.

You mustn't imagine that because your blood may be deficient in iron oxide you can go round to the druggist, buy some iron oxide, swallow it and cure yourself of this deficiency. It isn't as simple as that. Though the iron in your blood is chemically the same as that you can buy in a drugstore, it lacks something. We don't know what.

Get your druggist to make you up an "iron tonic," and it may make you feel better temporarily and give you an appetite, but the odds are that it will also make you constipated.

Feeding experiments with animals have shown that iron salts added to their feed destroy several important organic components of the diet. Ferrous sulfate, when added to their food, destroys vitamin A, and ferric chloride destroys vitamin E. This danger is always present when chemists think they know better than Nature.

Minerals Stored by the Body

There's some principle lacking in chemical iron that iron from living creatures contains and one day we may discover what it is. The grasses of the field possess the power to translate chemical iron, such as is found in the earth into substances that can be assimilated by Man and the lower animals.

One authority tells us that a man weighing 150 pounds carries in his body 90 pounds of oxygen, 36 pounds of carbon, 14 pounds of hydrogen, 3½ pounds of nitrogen, 3¾ pounds of calcium, 1 pound 14 ounces of phosphorus, 4 ounces of chlorine, 3½ ounces of sulfur, 3 ounces of potassium, 2½ ounces of sodium, 2 ounces of fluorine, 1½ ounces of magnesium, ¼ ounce of silicon, ⅙ ounce of iron.

In addition there are traces of nickel, cobalt and lead in the pancreas; tin in the suprenal capsules; zinc in the liver, kidneys, genital and other organs, and also in the thyroid glands; silver in the uterus, ovaries and thyroid, heart, spleen and kidneys; aluminum in lungs, kidneys, heart, testicles and pancreas; tin in all organs, but mainly in the brain, spleen and thyroid; copper in lungs, liver and heart, with traces in other organs; titanium in the lungs, with traces elsewhere.

All these play their part in the maintenance of health; if absent, one or more organs suffer. We have learned, for instance, that if cobalt is absent from the stomach the number of red blood corpuscles falls in number alarmingly and pernicious anemia develops.

What the result is of the absence of some of the other minerals, we do not as yet know; but we have found that in the case of cobalt a microscopic quantity makes all the difference between life and death.

Unless there is cobalt in the soil in which food is grown, vitamin B_{12} will not form in the stomach and without this vitamin the body cannot make use of iron. So, one falls a prey to anemia if either iron or cobalt is absent.

F. Newman Turner, a farmer renowned for his study of the soil and his desire to work with Nature rather than against her, found a cure for "staggers," a disease which affects cows put out to pasture after winter. The animals grow listless and ultimately collapse.

Mr. Turner, who owns a herd of disease-free Jersey cattle on his Wiltshire farm, thought that the disease was caused by mineral deficiency, so instead of plowing artificials into the soil he tried a "back-to-Nature-cure," by sowing deep-rooting herbs in his pastures.

Importance of Trace Elements

Other successful farmers like Friend Sykes and the late Louis Bromfield, who turned a wilderness in Ohio into one of the most flourishing farms in America, attest to the value of deep-rooting grasses. In *Out of the Earth* he gives a photograph of an alfalfa root which burrowed 15 feet into gravelly subsoil for its mineral diet.

Sugar cane is another deep-rooted grass and that, perhaps, is how it obtains the trace minerals which make molasses so valuable a food; that perhaps is why cane sugar smells and tastes so much more appetizing than beet sugar manufactured from a shallow-rooting tuber.

The thyroid glands remain inactive if iodine is missing and the result in babies is cretinism. Your body needs 75 micrograms of iodine a day—not very much when you learn that a microgram is one-thousandth part of a milligram; and that a milligram is a thousandth part of a gram, which weighs 3½ ounces. All the iodine your body needs every 24 hours is 75/1,000,000 parts of 3½ ounces. But, if it lacks that quantity, look out for trouble.

Both calcium and phosphorus are needed for bones and teeth, but the amount of calcium must be related to the amount of phosphorus in the body; and calcium cannot be used unless vitamin D is also present.

Once you embark on the study of food you realize that inside the body not only are foods interrelated with each other, but with vitamins, minerals, etc. No part of the human system is entirely and utterly independent of the others, though sometimes we imagine in our ignorance that some of them are.

Chlorine, which most of us consume as common salt, is needed for the manufacture of hydrochloric acid, a substance which breaks down proteins in the stomach and helps the blood to carry away waste products; and sodium is one of the main elements in tissue fluids throughout the body.

Magnesium and manganese are needed for bone growth and sulfur for skin and hair. Most proteins contain sulfur; so does vitamin B—but eggs, meat, fish and cereals are the best sources. Boil an egg until it is hard, cut it in half and around the yolk you will see a dark green layer of sulfur in combination with iron.

How aluminum arrives in the body we don't quite know, though aluminum cooking vessels doubtless throw off minute quantities into the food. But aluminum must be ingested by the eating of fruits, vegetables and flesh.

Arsenic is obtained possibly from oysters, flat fish and some fruits, such as peaches, the stones of which are rich in arsenic. Boron and copper exist in vegetables and fluoride in water. In some places there is so much fluorine in the water that it preserves the teeth of the population; in Pretoria and Madras such excess that it stiffens the joints, poisons the body, causes deformity of the spine and ossifies soft tissues!

The body contains nickel and silicon, too, but how they arrive and how they are replenished remains a mystery; nor do we know what happens if they are missing. We lack much knowledge about zinc as well. All we know is that if it is not present, diabetes develops.

Scientists interested in food and human welfare now realize that health starts in the soil, and if the earth in which plants are grown is devoid of minute traces of certain elements, specific diseases will overtake humans and animals who consume such produce. Some of these elements appear in such minute quantities in the soil, and even smaller quantities in food that they are known as "trace elements."

Countless thousands of dollars spent throughout the world, for instance, in cancer research, appear to lead nowhere. In 1954, however, the *British Journal of Cancer* published a significant report entitled "Soil Tests for Cancer," which revealed the information that in heavy cancer districts the copper supply of plants is much poorer than in districts where cancer is almost unknown. Perhaps —who knows?—copper in the soil may be part protection against the scourge.

Trees and plants sometimes suffer from a lack of zinc in the soil. Quite by accident a scientist stuck a zinc tack into an ailing tree—and cured it! This accident led to experiments which proved the need of plants for zinc.

Dr. E. V. McCollum, one of the greatest dietetic experts in the world, and famous for his discoveries in the vitamin field, found that if soil is deficient in manganese, the food grown in it will be deficient also.

Male rats fed on produce so deficient became sterile and female rats could produce no litters. Plants also suffered. Oats developed "grey speck," peas "march spot," and tomatoes lacked vitamin C; all because the soil in which they were grown lacked manganese.

Apples grown in soil deficient in boron were found to have spongy brown patches inside, and beets had "heart rot."

We are on the fringe of important discoveries in the field of farming and dietetics. There is so much we don't know about the growth of plants, animals and humans, but when eventually scientists unearth these secrets they may sweep many more illnesses from the world within a few years.

Among the foods which still arrive on our tables without being tampered with unnecessarily are molasses, black treacle and the richer forms of brown sugar.

They are grown in soil not heavily impregnated with artificial fertilizers; in fact, the soil in which sugar cane is grown is manured naturally, and so is that in which grow the various palms that produce jaggery.

And even if artificials were used, a deep-rooting grass like the cane would burrow far below into the subsoil to obtain essential ingredients from the rocks—the vast untapped storehouse of Nature.

Molasses is rich in vitamin B_1 or thiamine, which passes out of the body and has to be replenished daily. It has been found that refined sugars (white sugar in particular) exhaust the vitamin B_1 in the body and distort the calcium-phosphorus content. In the course of years this depletion can lead to serious consequences and result in diabetes, skin rashes, eye diseases, rheumatism, arthritis and sundry ailments.

Professor John Yudkin, of London University, stated recently that "Much of our present dietary trouble arises from the fact that 200 years ago Man learned to isolate sugar."* That is why you should always use either honey or molasses as a sweetener.

Incidentally, people badly afflicted by flies and midges in summer will find that if they give up sugar entirely, these creatures will no longer hanker after their blood!

* *Sunday Citizen*, November 18, 1962.

THE VITAMINS IN MOLASSES

MOLASSES and black treacle contain thiamine or vitamin B_1; riboflavin or B_2; nicotinic acid; B_6; pantothenic acid choline, and, according to Mark Dixon, traces of inositol have recently been isolated.

So many claims have been made for the miracles that molasses has achieved that one should not brush them aside without investigation. The fact that it contains so many vitamins of the B family makes it a valuable food.

We know a great deal about B_1, B_2, and nicotinic acid; something about B_6 and pantothenic acid, and a little about choline and inositol. These have been isolated only recently and there is still much research to be carried out.

Vitamin B_1 Essential to Health

B_1 is, fortunately, a vitamin which occurs in many foods; fortunately, because like vitamin C it passes out into the urine, is lost to the body and has to be replenished daily. If you don't have enough of it, all sorts of complications follow.

If your diet is a generous one embracing a wide variety of foods, you are bound to get a fair quota of vitamin B_1—but not, perhaps, as much as you should.

Your body needs 750–1,000 international units a day and a diet which includes a liberal amount of salads, fresh fruit, milk, cheese and meat will provide about 500. Wholemeal bread is a rich source of B_1, but how many eat 100 per cent wholemeal bread? The 85 per cent extraction flour from which "brown" bread can be baked is poor in B_1, containing less than one-third the amount found in wholemeal. As for white flour—it contains between a fifth and a quarter; and very fine, white, cake-and-pastry flour contains *no vitamin B_1 at all!*

There is a loaf in Britain which is made of 75 per cent white flour and 25 per cent wheat germ, which in theory should be an excellent source of B_1. Unfortunately, if kept, the wheat germ gets rancid, so in order to preserve it, the wheat germ is treated with superheated steam. "This," according to Professor Levine of the Rockefeller Institute, a great authority on B_1, "is no good. Vitamin B_1 is thermo-labile and superheated steam destroys it." Perhaps the bakers of this particular bread don't know.

The obvious question then is: "Why doesn't the B_1 in wholemeal bread get destroyed when subjected to baking?"

The answer is, of course, that though the oven may be 550 degrees F. when the loaf is put in, in ten minutes it falls to 500, and though a loaf may have been in the oven for forty-five minutes, the inside never reaches boiling point.

Incidentally, when I bake a loaf, the oven is never more than 350 degrees.

In view of the fact that so much bread that we believe has vitamin B_1 contains none at all, it is as well to make sure of getting enough by eating either brewer's yeast or some other food rich in the vitamin.

Brewer's yeast contains 500–700 I.U. of B_1 per ounce, and in powdered form is so light that a considerable amount would have to be swallowed. Few know about it, not many like it, though sprinkled on soups and salads it is palatable enough, and one doubts whether one person in a thousand stocks it in the larder. A pity, because it is an excellent protein food.

Peanut butter is another good source of B_1 for each ounce contains 125 I.U., and though you might like it on bread, how many could digest an

ounce of peanut butter every day? I know some
who like it but simply can't digest it.

So we fall back on molasses and black treacle. If
you eat a teaspoonful with porridge or wheat germ
at breakfast and another at night in either milk or
warm water, you will go a long way to making up
any deficiency of B_1.

There are so many ways in which both can be
eaten: on bread, with milk or water, with or without the addition of lemon; in cakes, puddings, tarts
and sweets, and made into toffee.

Their value is increased as foods because both
are so palatable that children like them, whereas
children don't much care for yeast. According to
C. C. and F. M. Furnas, authorities on diet, "sul-
phur-and-molasses wasn't bad medicine for children, *if the molasses was black.*" It contained pre-
cious iron and Vitamin B.

What happens if your body lacks B_1?

If the deficiency is severe as it sometimes still is
with thousands of undernourished people in Asia,
Africa and South America and in remote areas of
Newfoundland and Labrador, then the victims
suffer from a form of neuritis or general weakness
known as beri-beri or polyneuritis. There are even
some in the hearts of great cities like New York,
Paris and London who enjoy ample incomes, live in
the midst of plenty and yet suffer from mild forms
of neuritis simply because they live on the wrong
foods, for malnutrition *is not necessarily* a disease
of the poor.

If the symptoms are severe, such people consult
a doctor or go into a hospital, but in mild forms of
neuritis they imagine they are suffering from "general debility," a phrase which covers a multitude of
ills, and take tonics or a change of air, which sometimes helps to alleviate because with it goes a
change of diet, too.

Everywhere one sees people who appear to be
"fat and healthy" (a contradiction of terms), but

possess neither energy nor stamina. This is usually because white sugar, white bread and cakes, buns and biscuits made from these comprise the bulk of their diet. They stream with chronic colds, for which their doctors have fancy names such as sinusitis or hay fever, and take pills by the score and potions by the gallon to rid them of their ailments.

Whereas, all they have to do is to throw the white flour and white sugar and everything that is made from them out of the window, and eat only dark brown sugar, 100 per cent wholemeal flour, molasses and black treacle.

B_1 is a nerve food. A lack of the vitamin weakens the nerves and makes them less responsive. If the shortage of B_1 is severe the nerves become crippled and the entire bodily mechanism is brought to a halt. In short, paralysis is the result.

This, of course, is only in cases of extreme deficiency. In *About Vitamins* I have cited the case of the islanders of Nauru who were struck down by polio because their food was deficient in B_1. In South India, for instance, millions who once ate rice coated with the thin red husk now eat only polished rice because Europeans eat it and it is the thing to do. They also spurn country-made jaggery and use refined sugar in its stead. As the South is a rice- and not bread-eating country, hundreds of thousands of women are feeling the effects of B_1 starvation.

Premature births in the South are three times as numerous as in the North. The women suffer from "neuritis of pregnancy," a disease which also afflicts millions in the U.S.A. and in Kashmir.

Dr. Kathleen Vaughan says, "Anemia is always present [among the well-to-do women of Kashmir] and unfortunately is admired," as it was in Victorian England, "as a fair complexion is a sign of being well-bred." They guard themselves from the sun and wear "burkas" (cloaks covering the head and body, with two lattice-holes for the eyes), eat refined food, and many also take arsenic to induce a pale complexion. This is started early and the doses are gradually increased, until some Kashmiri women gain such tolerance for the poison that they can take enough arsenic to kill any European. All in aid of beauty!

B_1 has in common with vitamin C the power to build stamina. Wherever men or women do a great deal of hard work, as in lumber camps and harvest fields, do overtime in factories or stand long hours over a washtub, there is an increase of metabolism (metabolism is the total of the chemical and physical changes which go on in the body, is estimated by measuring the rate at which oxygen is used, and defined in calories, or the amount of heat produced) which calls for an increase of vitamin B_1. If this need is not met over an appreciable length of time the victims fall ill with fevers—hyperthyroidism.

This necessary addition to diet is overlooked when troops are sent on long, arduous expeditions simply because the knowledge of the authorities lags behind the findings of scientists. Nurses who work extra hours during epidemics carry on in health because the mind drives one in a crisis, but when the crisis is over there is a reaction and collapse.

Scientific expeditions, like those to the Poles and Mount Everest, have taught us a good deal. Both Shackleton and Donald B. MacMillan, leader of the Croaker Land Expedition 1913–17, learned from the disasters of others.

"I was with Peary on his trip to the North Pole in 1909," wrote MacMillan, "when it was the common experience of all of us to suffer from bleeding intestines.

"Peary believed in beef, suet, raisins, tea, ships biscuits (*white flour*) and condensed milk." Peary took 10,000 pounds of *white flour*, 1,000 of coffee,

800 of tea, 10,000 of *white sugar*, 7,000 of bacon, 10,000 of *white* biscuit, 30,000 of pemmican, 3,000 of dried fish, and 10,000 cans of condensed milk.

MacMillan took *wholemeal* biscuits, *wholemeal* flour, dehydrated vegetables (potatoes, rhubarb, turnips, spinach, onions), dehydrated soup, yellow-eyed beans, pea beans, Scotch green peas, yellow split peas, dried apples and apricots, prunes, raisins, chocolate (both bitter and sweet), *brown sugar*, baked beans, nuts, dates, figs, lime juice, cherries, plums, corn, peas, tomatoes and squash.

They lived on these foods for four years and returned without any sign of scurvy or other deficiency diseases.

Shackleton says in *Heart of the Antarctic:* "In the first place food must be wholesome and nourishing in the highest degree. At one time the dread scurvy disease was regarded as the inevitable result of a prolonged stay in ice-bound regions, and even the *Discovery* Expedition during its labors in the Antarctic, 1902–1904, suffered from scurvy, but during our entire trip from 1907 to 1909 we did not develop a single case of the sickness, relying almost exclusively on *whole wheat* biscuit, dehydrated fruits and vegetables, marrowfat peas, lentils and kidney beans.

"We carried with us dried prunes, peaches, apricots, raisins, currants, apples, dehydrated potatoes, carrots, cabbage, onions, Brussels sprouts, cauliflower, celery, spinach, parsley, mint, rhubarb, mushrooms and artichokes to the extent of 3,800 pounds, with 2,240 pounds, of *whole wheat* biscuit."

Unhappily, Scott's ill-fated expedition three years later did not apply this knowledge.

Molasses isn't mentioned, but MacMillan took *brown* sugar, which is the next best thing. Both expeditions stressed the value of *wholemeal* flour and biscuit, which contain B_1.

B_1 gives you staying power; that is why brown bread is so much more satisfying that white; why brown sugar is a food whereas white is a poison; why molasses and black treacle are so good for you.

Earlier I referred to the brimstone and treacle which children years ago were made to take in the spring "to clear the blood." How it actually worked, our grandfathers did not know, but Dr. L. J. Picton, in *Thoughts on Feeding*, says: "Vitamin B_1 is rich in sulphur and is the only vitamin so far known to contain that element."

Picton relates the case of an old lady who ate little else but white bread five times a day, along with tea. She fell ill with beri-beri; her heart muscle was loaded with lactic as well as pyruvic acid and as a result she developed a craving for onions, which are rich in sulfur. "I wonder," Picton remarks, "whether the sulfur had anything to do with the *aneurin* (B_1) which in the old lady's case had been so long absent, and somehow helped to clear the lactic and pyruvic acids which were blocking the cardiac muscles?"

Constipation is a Disease

One of our worst modern diseases is constipation, though people don't think about it as a disease because, except in extreme forms, it can be relieved, but not cured, by laxatives. Advice in the form of advertisements abounds, and it is so much easier to take a pill, a dose of "fruit salts" (which have no fruit essences whatever in them), or a chocolate-coated tablet.

But these are, at best, only palliatives, and will never cure. In order that your bowels will evacuate the residue from food after the nutriment has been extracted from it, your diet must contain vitamins of the B complex, especially B_1, as well as a certain amount of roughage usually in the form of cellulose from greenstuff and fruit.

All authoritative medical writers agree that constipation is a disease of civilization and that among savages constipation is unknown. Most people regard it as a normal state, and when they shop at weekends millions of housewives budget for laxatives. Constipation starts in infancy and the most common cause is the abuse of purgatives in infancy: castor oil and soap-and-water enemas. "These methods," says Dr. Eric Pritchard in *The Physiological Feeding of Infants and Children*, "are usually regarded as harmless and efficacious . . . all of them are, however, in my experience prolific causes of chronic constipation." He adds: "The regular taking of laxatives has become so deeply ingrained in the majority of us, and even in doctors, midwives and nurses, that the unfortunate baby, though born healthy and normal, is promptly dosed with aperients as if it were crippled in health and suffered from chronic constipation."

What is the result of taking laxatives regularly? The bowel becomes lazy; it has no work to do, and eventually when called upon to function, it cannot.

Palliatives at best; that is what laxatives are. They never cure, though they are invaluable in emergencies.

When filled with rough residue which they can grip, the muscles of the bowels have a gentle, massaging movement, like waves, called peristaltic action. The action keeps on, day and night, without any effort on your part—and it may continue for some time after death.

Alvarez, the great American physiologist, who worked with the Mayo brothers at their famous clinic in Rochester, Minnesota, cut out a frog's stomach and placed it in a salt solution, and long after the frog was dead the waves of stomach movement continued.

Dr. Henry Borsook says that a mild vitamin B_1 deficiency will cause constipation, flatulence and dyspepsia in middle and old age, and hand in hand with these symptoms go headaches, lack of stamina and chronic fatigue. He remarks that unless there is an ulcer, tumor or other infection, these conditions can be cured by a daily supplement of 750–1,000 I.U. of vitamin B complex.

Middle and old age are specifically mentioned because in youth, when one is extremely active, hard exercise often cures constipation, despite the wrong diet. Especially swimming in which the stomach muscles are given a great deal of work, though we don't realize it.

In 1932 M. S. Rose and his associates McLeod, Vahlteich, Funnell and Newton carried out experiments and wrote a treatise: *The Influence of Bran on the Alimentary Canal,* in which they showed that vitamin B_1 has a beneficial effect on gastrointestinal functions and corrects many types of constipation. They found that not only the bulk of bran but its vitamin content helped, and that wheat germ, too, was effective in cases of constipation.

It should be made a crime against the people to make bread from flour from which the bran or the wheat germ has been removed, and then to sell that bran at an inflated price as a "health food."

The All-Bran on sale in shops is slightly sweet; it is usually mixed with molasses.

The late Mahatma Gandhi, who was a great exponent of healthy living and wrote a book on "Diet Reform," realized that all-bran as sold in England and America, was much too costly for the millions of poor in India, so on the advice of Dr. W. R. Ackroyd, he advised them to buy bran sold very cheaply as cattle food and mix it with either jaggery or molasses.

In Britain bran can be bought at six cents a pound, and two teaspoons of bran can be converted into a wholesome and palatable breakfast food with the addition of a teaspoon of molasses or black treacle and warm milk. It is preferable to the patented article, which undergoes heat treatment.

Both honey and molasses are very good foods for

the heart. "Heart disease" is an extremely loose term embracing all sorts of heart conditions. Where neuritis is associated with an enlargement of the heart there is usually a vitamin B_1 deficiency and in such cases molasses or black treacle will work wonders. Either can be taken mixed in warm water. The alternative is, on a doctor's orders, to take B_1 in capsule form—10–50 milligrams daily—though it is preferable by far to take foods containing vitamins than capsules in which synthetic vitamins are imprisoned.

As a principle the pill habit should be shunned.

Dr. Arthur Goulston says in his book *Sugar Cane and Heart Disease* that malnutrition of the heart vessel is a common cause of heart failure and is responsible, in fact, for far more heart failures than one suspects.

"Failure is accompanied by a state known as auricular fibrillation, characterized by very rapid beat."

He recommends levulose as the necessary activator in such cases and adds *"The nearer we get to the sugar cane*, the more activator we shall get," which means either pure sugar cane sap, unobtainable commercially, or the edibles closest to it—molasses, black treacle and thick, rich, brown sugar.

In such cases the heart needs its own weight in sap daily; that is, about 8–9 ounces. According to *The Medical Annual*, 8 ounces of cane sap have been given every 24 hours, with astonishing results.

This treatment is based on the need of the heart for glycogen; that the best source of glycogen is levulose; and the best sources of levulose are honey, pure cane sap, molasses, black treacle and rich brown sugar.

When dentists inveigh against sugar, what they refer to is *refined sugar*. Dr. F. A. Sterling of New York declared: "Natives of Africa whom I have examined have possessed teeth in perfect condition, due entirely to their living on coarse, natural foods. I have observed that the nearer people are to primitive nature, the better their teeth. The colored race, particularly those living on whole corn meal and the *unrefined sugar cane* diet of the southern plantations, have good teeth."

Dr. J. Archambeau, also of New York, endorses this. "The people of the British West Indies subsist on yams, vegetables, bananas, *sugar cane in abundance*, a little salt fish and very little meat. Decayed teeth are very rare. Most of their teeth look as if they were fashioned from ivory."

Why? Because, as Professor J. C. Drummond says: "There is present in whole wheat meal, whole maize sugar, crude sugar-cane juice . . . a substance which protects the surface of the teeth from the action of fermenting material produced in the crevices. This protective substance is lost when flour is refined to give a 'high-grade' white product, or when sugar is converted into the 'clean, pure' material we use nowadays at table."

Riboflavin or B₂

Riboflavin or B_2, another invaluable member of the vitamin B family, is found in abundance in yeast, the bran and germ of wheat, molasses, black treacle, brown sugar, beer and tea. Beer is not the best recommended source, and the amount in tea is small.

Its main contribution is to the health of the eyes. Once it was thought that if vitamin A were missing the eyes would be affected and night-blindness ensue. But it was found that some cases of glare-blindness do not respond to A, but to B_2, and soon research in this direction was pursued.

There are no blood vessels in the cornea of the eye for those which sprout from the conjunctiva normally cease to spread when they reach the junction of the cornea and the sclera, or white of the eye. But if there is a deficiency of riboflavin in the system the blood vessels from the conjunctiva invade the cornea and may even encroach into the area of the pupil. Opaque spots then appear in the cornea and the eyes grow sore and inflamed.

Within recent years there has been abundant evidence that riboflavin is necessary for eye health, and in experiments, animals deprived of riboflavin have grown cataracts.

Vitamin B is also needed for the nerves— especially the nerves of the eye when diseased by heavy drinking and smoking.

One hospital approached ten alcohol amblyopias and offered them free board and lodging as well as unlimited booze and tobacco if they would submit to treatment by B complex vitamins. The bait was so succulent that they swallowed it and nine were completely cured! The tenth was too far gone. The patients must have had a really gay time for one gentleman consumed as much as a quart of whiskey a day—which speaks volumes for the potency of B complex!

B_2 is far less affected by heat than B_1; on the other hand, like vitamin C it is destroyed both by visible and ultraviolet light.

Nicotinic Acid or P-P; also called Niacin

Another important member of the B family is nicotinic acid, sometimes called P-P, or Pellagra Preventive, because if the system lacks P-P you will fall a victim to pellagra, a dreadful deficiency disease once confused with beri-beri.

It was thought in America where millions of poor whites in the South suffered from pellagra, that this affliction was caused by the three M's— Meat, Maize and Molasses. The meat eaten was usually salt pork; the maize was husked; the molasses was not really molasses at all, but a syrup denuded of all minerals. No one can exist in health on such a diet and investigations proved that they existed on the worst kind of refined-food diet possible.

In his *Science of Eating*, Alfred W. McCann says: "Commercial molasses represents the liquid that remains after the extraction of the first, second and third crop of sugar and the addition of the chemicals necessary to the extraction, including sulfites.

"The stuff known as 'first molasses' contains what is left of the cane syrup after a single crop of crystalline sugar has been extracted." It can be seen from this that the "molasses" eaten in the South has no connection with the molasses recommended by dietitians.

The Federal Writers' Project published a number of brief biographies ("These Are Our Lives") issued by the University of North Carolina Press, throwing a vivid light on the way they lived and ate. One writer describes his father returning home late in the evening, dog-tired and "eatin' our scant meal of cornbread, peas and cane sirup," a syrup denuded of all minerals.

Like all deficiency diseases caused by a lack of the B complex, pellagra ultimately destroys the nervous system and the end is insanity and death.

During the first world war soldiers in the trenches contracted what is known as "trench mouth," a mild form of pellagra due to an endless diet of bully beef, biscuits and bread made of white flour, strong tea sweetened with white sugar, and plum and apple jam. Only when thousands fell ill and a manpower crisis became imminent did the authorities add dehydrated vegetables and other comestibles to their impoverished diet.

There are many foods rich in one or other of the B complex vitamins: brewer's yeast, wholemeal flour, liver, kidney, oysters, mutton, beef (a little), molasses, *but none in white sugar*.

The other B vitamins mentioned by Hauser and Marc Dixon as being present in molasses are B_6, an anti-gray-hair filtrate, pantothenic acid, choline and inositol.

B_6 was known at first as adermin, now as pyridoxine and was isolated in 1938. Experiments have proved that a deficiency of this vitamin in rats results in diseases of the skin and hair; in dogs, anemia, but when used in conjunction with B_1 and B_2 and E, has proved of value in the treatment of certain degenerative diseases of the human nervous system.

Crude molasses is the best known source of B_6 but *beet molasses contains none at all*. This may be because sugar cane is a deep-rooting grass which absorbs sulfur and other chemicals from deep down in the soil. Beet, with shallow roots, does not. The bran of cereals is a good source of B_6; fish and meat, fair; fruits and vegetables, poor; seeds, legumes and cereals, the best known sources.

Much has yet to be learned about B_6 and there is little point in making extravagant claims on its behalf, which cannot be proved.

Anti-gray-hair filtrate. The gray-haired and balding roués needn't imagine that something has been discovered that will return such of their locks as remain to their pristine hue. But—there is hope. In 1930 Professor Gabriel Bertrand of the Academy of Sciences in Paris noted that three biologists in his laboratory fed gray-haired rats on synthetic vitamins of the B family, and their coats turned black!

But they didn't think the discovery was worth following up. In 1938 Dr. Agnes Fay Morgan of the Department of Household Science at the University of California made a similar observation, but in another way. She became interested in a vitamin B_2 filtrate factor, discovered by Drs. T. H. Jukes and F. Lepkovsky, while experimenting with chickens. They found this factor essential to the life and growth of chickens and told Dr. Morgan about it.

Dr. Morgan was interested, not in turning gray hair black, but in curing cataract, but she found that when rats with cataract were fed with vitamin B_2 filtrate factor, their gray hair turned black after only 8–12 weeks.

She experimented with rats because their life span is roughly three years, and it was mainly with three-year-old rats, corresponding to humans aged ninety, that she worked. If this filtrate factor acts on humans as it does on rats, it will give a tremendous boost to all gray-haired people—especially women, some of whom spend small fortunes on dyes.

There is no reason why it shouldn't for there are instances of explorers—notably Adolphus W. Greely—who have been away from civilization, lived on denatured foods for two or three years and returned looking old, emaciated and gray. Dr. Greely's hair was almost entirely gray when he returned from an Arctic expedition, but six months on food rich in B vitamins restored it to its natural color.

Strong emotion, such as anxiety and shock, also tend to turn the hair gray. Historians tell us that both Marie Antoinette and Mary Queen of Scots turned gray while in prison awaiting execution, and there are many other examples, A Miss Knowles, headmistress of Queen's Hill School, Darjeeling, India, whose school was involved in a landslide disaster, turned gray overnight because of the anxiety she experienced over her charges.

Apparently melanin, the coloring matter in hair, is affected by nervous stress—and B_2, contained in molasses and black treacle, is good for the nerves.

Choline

There is some doubt whether choline can be classified as a vitamin, for substitutes that are not vitamins can be used instead, such as menthionine (an amino acid) and betaine (chemically related to an amino acid). It doesn't really matter whether it is a vitamin or not. Amino acids, incidentally, are the building blocks from which proteins are formed.

All this might be somewhat too technical for the layman, so to put it into plain terms, choline and inositol are substances that keep fat on the move and prevent it from adhering to the walls of the arteries.

If there is a deficiency of choline in the system the liver becomes clogged with fat, leading to cirrhosis of the liver; the kidneys bleed (hemorrhage of the kidneys); and the body may become paralyzed or develop abnormalities.

Fatty liver is caused by the failure of the mobilization of the *methyl groups;* this interferes with the transport of fat, causing it to accumulate on the liver.

If your diet is excessively rich in fat, choline is an essential ingredient; but if it contains a preponderance of protein, such as casein, which contains a good deal of menthionine, then you don't need so much choline. Excessive protein can lead, however, to troubles of its own.

It has been found that a lack of choline in chickens causes *perosis* or slipped tendon, though we don't know about other of its effects upon humans.

In hospitals choline is given to patients where excessive wastage of protein is apparent, as in cases of scalds, burns, severe wounds and high fevers; and where doctors have found diets excessively rich in protein, food containing choline is advised. *Among the richest sources are molasses*, which has 290 milligrams to the pound, and *black treacle*.

Arteriosclerosis, or hardening of the arteries, usually caused by rich feeding and extreme pressure of work, is a disease which takes toll of millions, and because directors of successful concerns work hard and are forced by circumstances to indulge in heavy luncheons, it is sometimes called "directors' disease."

For years we have been told that one of the main causes is too much fat in food. Olive oil is one of the few edible fats that does NOT tend to bring about arteriosclerosis, but few, apart from those who live in the Mediterranean area, eat or cook with olive oil.

Richard Yaffe, who has written an authoritative book on the subject, says that arteriosclerosis affects about 26 per cent of those between 40–49; 48 per cent between 50–59; and 90 per cent of those who are 90 and over—at which age it doesn't really matter very much.

The villain of the piece is a fatty substance called cholesterol, which combines with other substances in the bloodstream and so thickens that it is unable to filter through the walls of the arteries and remains embedded in them.

When this happens, calcium starts to deposit and thicken on these blocks and the arteries become hard, rigid, unreceptive and prevent nourishment from seeping through.

If this continues long enough a host of unpleasant symptoms arise, among them loss of memory and inability to concentrate, high blood pressure and giddiness, and if diet and the way of life are not altered drastically death will probably follow.

Cholesterol is a necessary ingredient of the body; only when there's an excess and when cholesterol starts choking the arteries does trouble start.

In parts of India and Southeast Asia, where people live on a low-fat diet, arteriosclerosis is unknown. Incidentally, these races also consume a good deal of jaggery or products made from pure cane syrup, and we have only recently realized that there is a distinct link between freedom from hardening of the arteries and molasses.

Inositol

Molasses and black treacle are also the richest sources of inositol, another substance which dissolves the fatty particles in the arteries and keeps them on the move. Very little about it is known, but Dr. Leslie J. Harris says in *Vitamins in Theory and Practice*, "As to its pro-vitamin properties, mice deprived of inositol are said to develop baldness. In rats a similar condition, a denuding of the hair around the eyes—picturesquely known as *spectacle eyes*—has been described."

This does not mean that the converse is true and that inositol added to the diet will produce hair. But there is always hope. And if with mice, why not humans?

Philip H. Van Itallie says in a paper entitled *Arteriosclerosis*, "It is virtually impossible to arrange a practical diet adequate for the body's reasonable needs without including, willy-nilly, some cholesterol. But there is a wide chasm between a scientific diet and the diet habitually consumed by most Americans.

"If all persons over forty were literally to go on a low-fat diet—an utterly fantastic supposition despite its scientific merits—the effect on the daily lives of Americans would be revolutionary."

The same applies also to people in Britain, Holland, Germany, Austria and the Scandinavian countries where immense quantities of fat are consumed as a buffer against the cold.

It's no use telling people that if they cut down on egg yolk, liver, kidney, heart, sweetbreads, oysters, fish roe, lard, fatty fish and animal fats of all kinds, including milk and cream, their chances of living to an old age will be rosier.

"A short life and a merry one," is what most people prefer, though unfortunately, life though often short is frequently the reverse of merry. People in general won't exclude fatty meat and shun gravy and gland-meats, such as liver, brain, etc.

Although this book has told you something about the virtues and curative properties of molasses and black treacle, don't run away with the idea that you can eat an abundance of foods that are bad for you, live "the life of Riley" and maintain excellent health and vigor by taking a few spoons of molasses daily.

You can't—though there are exceptions to every rule. Some are endowed by Nature with iron constitutions which enable them to break every rule of health and get away with it. Such are few and far between.

A balanced diet and sane, *moderate* living is the only sure path to health. I have elsewhere quoted E. V. McCollum, the famous scientist and dietitian, as saying that if only all people ate like the French they would have little need to worry about diet sheets. In France it is tradition to finish every substantial meal with a salad, and Escoffier, the renowned chef, devised a variety of salads to be eaten after hot roasts.

In France, too (though not perhaps in Paris), a good deal of 100 per cent wholemeal bread is consumed; far more than in either Britain or America. Not because books tell the French to do so but because their sturdy ancestors loved such bread. And the average working-class French housewife buys a far wider variety of foods than her English counterpart. One has merely to visit a French market to confirm this.

This variety ensures that all the essential minerals and vitamins are included.

Many apparently miraculous cures have been wrought by people who maintain that they have taken molasses or black treacle regularly, but in the light of common sense it would be a trifle ingenuous to believe that either molasses or black treacle are magical elixirs or panaceas that will banish all ills.

Each time you learn of a case in which molasses or treacle has wrought a miracle, examine it and find out whether the sufferer was as ill as made out, what changes were made in his regimen, and other details, and the odds are that you will discover that an all-round change has been made in his way of living: diet, rest, possibly a change of environment or a short fast.

Molasses isn't magic. It can do just so much and no more.

You must work WITH NATURE, not AGAINST her.

Molasses and treacle are foods that make up deficiencies in diet lacking certain substances; they are not complete foods in themselves, complete in the sense that they alone will furnish the body with all it needs.

In *Man, Bread and Destiny*, the Furnas brothers say: "The main shortages in our average national [American] dietary seem to be those of iron, calcium and vitamins A, C and G (this is B_2 or riboflavin, sometimes called G in honor of Joseph Goldberger, who thought it would cure pellagra). Molasses and black treacle are rich in iron, calcium and G."

The average British diet is certainly short of some of the B-complex vitamins, possibly calcium and iron, and because of the lack of sunshine, perhaps vitamin D. Here again, molasses and treacle can be taken with benefit by almost anyone. But to claim that they can cure a variety of virulent diseases would be dishonest.

In our little village lives an eminent Roman Catholic priest known for his scientific activities. Though I am not of his flock, he and I are good friends.

Before coming here he labored so hard that he fell ill with high blood pressure, hardening of the arteries and other complications. The mere effort of bending to tie his shoelaces made his temples throb and his heart thump like a pile driver. He couldn't walk up even a short flight of stairs, and the mere effort of speaking exhausted him. His days in the ministry, if not on earth, seemed numbered.

Eventually he fell into the hands of someone who specialized in health rather than disease, and was persuaded to take a short fast. His diet was radically changed and his entire life reorganized. Instead of rich meats and red wines he ate salads and drank water. White bread, white flour and white sugar were banished from his household and replaced by wholemeal flour and rich brown sugar. Honey and molasses were introduced into his diet and gradually he grew fitter and stronger.

Today at sixty he cycles and walks miles. He has charge of the souls of people in a number of parishes and is one of the most energetic men I know. Recently he was examined and no sign could be found of high blood pressure. The learned specialist who conducted the test said that our priest has the arteries of a young man and expressed astonishment that at his age he could be cured so thoroughly.

Needless to say, our priest now swears not only by honey and molasses but by every item of his changed diet.

It would be true to say that many who were extremely ill—even at death's door—have been cured by an entire change of diet and helped on the way back to health by such foods as molasses, black treacle, honey, yeast, wheat germ, yogurt, and the vitamins, mineral salts and acids in fresh vegetables and fruit.

One has only to read that inspiring book *Crude Black Molasses* by Cyril Scott to realize just how much good molasses can do.

MOLASSES RECIPES

N.B. *Where wholemeal flour is mentioned, always buy a well-known make. There are many on the market and if you can't buy such flour from your grocer, get it at one of the numerous Health Food Stores.*

The best known makes of 100-per-cent wholemeal flour contain wheat grown in compost, and tends to build up bodily resistance against disease.

For recipes requiring salt, sea or biochemic salt only should be used. When sugar is listed as an ingredient, always use unrefined brown sugar such as Barbados.

A good breakfast dish can be made with:

1 tablespoon breakfast cereal (optional)
1 tablespoon wheat germ
2 teaspoons pure bran
1 teaspoon molasses or black treacle
Enough warm or cold milk to cover the ingredients, or perhaps a little more.

Instead of the breakfast cereal, try "coarse oats." Coarse oats are much better food than rolled oats, because when rolled some of the natural fat is squeezed out and lost. Cover the coarse oats with boiling or very hot milk overnight and allow them to soak. Next morning they will be soft enough to chew and so give the teeth the exercise they need, and the treacle will render the mixture palatable. Too much molasses or treacle is liable to sicken children of this excellent food.

Coarse oats also provide more mineral matter than either rolled oats or oatmeal. In this dish your child will get carbohydrate, vitamins E, B complex, A and D, and some calcium and phosphorus.

MOLASSES BRAN BREAD
   1 teaspoon soda
   ½ cup molasses
   1½ cups sour milk (or yogurt)
   1½ cups wholemeal flour
   1½ cups bran
   ½ cup seeded raisins

Dissolve soda in molasses, add milk, flour, bran and raisins. Bake for 45 minutes in moderate over (350 degrees Fahrenheit) in a loaf pan. This may be baked in smaller molds.

DATE BRAN BREAD
   ½ cup molasses
   1 egg
   1 cup milk
   1½ cups bran
   2 cups wholemeal flour
   ⅛ teaspoon soda
   1 tablespoon baking powder
   ½ teaspoon salt
   2 tablespoons melted shortening
   ½ cup chopped dates

Mix the molasses, egg and milk. Add the dry ingredients mixed together. Then add the melted shortening and dates. Bake in a medium-sized bread pan for 45 minutes in a moderate oven. Raisins may be substituted for dates.

MOLASSES ORANGE BREAD
   ½ cup sugar
   2⅔ cups wholemeal flour
   ½ teaspoon baking soda
   2 teaspoons baking powder
   1½ teaspoons salt
   ⅔ cup milk
   1 tablespoon grated orange rind
   ½ cup orange juice
   2 tablespoons salad oil
   ½ cup molasses
   1 cup chopped nuts or raisins

Sift together sugar, flour, baking soda, baking powder and salt. Add nuts or raisins. Combine milk, orange rind, orange juice, salad oil and molasses. Add to flour mixture all at once; stir just enough to blend. Turn into well greased loaf pan 9 x 5 x 2¾ inches. Bake in slow oven at 325 degrees Fahrenheit for 1¼ hours. Cool before removing from pan.

TROPICAL GINGERBREAD
½ cup butter
½ cup sugar
2 eggs
1 teaspoon soda
½ cup molasses
1 teaspoon ginger
1 teaspoon cinnamon
¼ teaspoon salt
1½ cups wholemeal flour
½ cup cold water
2 cups freshly grated or moist-packed coconut

Cream butter and sugar well, add eggs and beat all together. Dissolve soda in molasses and add to first mixture. Mix and sift remaining dry ingredients, adding to first mixture alternately with the cold water. Stir in 1 cup of the coconut. Pour into well-greased pan and bake in moderate oven at 350 degrees Fahrenheit for 35 minutes. Ice with a frosting made as follows: Boil 1 cup sugar and ¼ cup water without stirring until syrup forms a long thread when dropped from spoon. Beat 2 egg whites stiff; pour syrup slowly over egg whites, stirring constantly. Add ¾ teaspoon lemon extract. Beat until right consistency to spread. Sprinkle thickly with remaining coconut.

STEAMED GINGER PUDDING
½ cup honey
1 tablespoon molasses
½ tablespoon melted shortening
½ cup sour milk or yogurt
1¾ cups self-rising wholemeal flour
½ teaspoon salt (optional)
1 teaspoon ginger

Sift together the dry ingredients; then add the melted shortening and beat well into them. Pour in the milk or yogurt, mix well and transfer to a well-greased mold and steam for 50–60 minutes. Some like this served with sliced oranges or orange juice, but try it plain, first.

STEAMED BERRY PUDDING

Use the same recipe for ginger pudding, but omit the ginger and substitute half a teaspoon of ground cloves and three-quarters of a teaspoon of ground cinnamon. Add a cup of any berries in season, and proceed as for the ginger pudding.

COCONUT PUDDING

3 cups milk
1 cup honey
2 tablespoons molasses
½ cup shredded coconut
1½ tablespoons tapioca or semolina
2½ tablespoons cornmeal
1 teaspoon salt (optional)

A few drops of real vanilla or 1 teaspoon lemon juice. Alternatively, grate the rind of one lemon.

I don't like adding salt to any recipe and sweet puddings are all the better without the addition of salt.

Scald the milk, mix all the remaining ingredients and stir them into the milk. Cook over hot water or in a double boiler till the mixture thickens slightly, then turn into a well-greased pudding dish and bake for 2 hours in a slow oven (250 degrees Fahrenheit), keeping the mixture covered for an hour and a half, then uncovering it for the last half-hour, to brown. Serve hot with cream or beaten yogurt.

THREE - INGREDIENTS - CAKE (Honey-apple molasses)

1½ cups thinly sliced apple
¾ cup honey
2 tablespoons molasses
½ cup hot water
2½ cups self-rising wholemeal flour
½ cup brown sugar
1 teaspoon ground cinnamon
½ teaspoon ground cloves
¼ teaspoon grated nutmeg
¼ teaspoon salt (optional)
⅓ cup shortening

Mix the honey and molasses; fold in the apples and cook on a low flame until they are tender. Then cool.

Now melt the shortening in hot water and mix it gradually into the flour, then add to all the other dry ingredients, little by little, constantly stirring to keep smooth. Finally stir in the honey-apple-molasses mixture. Pour into a shallow greased dish and bake in a moderate oven for 45–60 minutes.

EGGLESS AND SUGARLESS CAKE

2½ cups self-rising wholemeal flour
1 cup sour milk or yogurt
1 cup honey
2 tablespoons molasses
2 teaspoons ginger
1 teaspoon ground cinnamon
½ teaspoon ground cloves
¼ cup shortening
½ teaspoon salt (optional)

Add the milk or yogurt to the honey and molasses. Sift the dry ingredients together and add them to the honey-yogurt-molasses. Then melt the shortening and add that. Beat vigorously. Pour into a greased shallow dish and bake in a moderate oven for 45 minutes.

MOLASSES CANDY

- ½ cup molasses
- ½ cup honey
- ½ cup peanut butter
- 1 cup powdered skim milk
- ½ cup seedless raisins or sultanas

Place the ingredients in a bowl and mix well. Then place the mixture on a board or enamel-top table, add more powdered skim milk until it is stiff and knead it. Continue to knead until the mixture is very stiff; then cut it into square or other convenient shapes and roll it in powdered brown sugar and cinnamon, or in shredded coconut.

As a sweet it is wholesome and nutritious and infinitely preferable to the concoctions sold in shops and made with either white sugar or glucose.

In these recipes honey is added to molasses or treacle, otherwise the treacly taste might pall.

GINGER NUTS

- 3 cups wholemeal flour
- 1 cup chopped raisins
- 1 teaspoon cinnamon
- ½ teaspoon cloves
- ½ teaspoon ginger
- ½ teaspoon salt
- ½ cup sugar
- ½ teaspoon soda
- ½ cup molasses
- 1 egg (beaten)
- ½ cup melted shortening

Mix and sift the dry ingredients. Add the molasses, egg and shortening. Mix to stiff dough. Shape in a long roll ¾ inch in diameter. Cut off ¾-inch pieces and roll in tiny balls. Roll each in sugar and bake in a moderate oven.

PLANTATION CUP CAKES

½ cup shortening
½ cup sugar
½ cup molasses
2 eggs
1½ cups wholemeal flour
¼ teaspoon soda
2 teaspoons baking powder
1 teaspoon cinnamon
¼ teaspoon mace
½ teaspoon salt
½ cup milk

Cream shortening and sugar together. Add the molasses and well-beaten eggs. Mix and sift dry ingredients, adding them alternately with the milk. Mix well. Bake in muffin pans in a hot oven for 20 minutes.

BROWNIES

⅔ cup sugar
⅔ cup shortening
¾ cup molasses
4 eggs
2 cups wholemeal flour
2 cups nuts (cut fine)

Cream the sugar and shortening, add the eggs and molasses, then the flour and nuts. Bake in a square or oblong pan and cut into squares. This will make about 3 dozen.